Book 1:

Coconut Oil for Skin Care & Hair Loss

&

Book 2:

Oil Pulling Therapy For Beginners

&

Book 3:

Healing Babies and Children with Aromatherapy for Beginners

Coconut Oil for Skin Care & Hair Loss

BY LINDSEY PYLARINOS

A Step by Step Guide for Using Virgin Coconut Oil for Youthful Skin and Healthy Hair

COCONUT OIL
FOR
SKIN CARE & HAIR LOSS

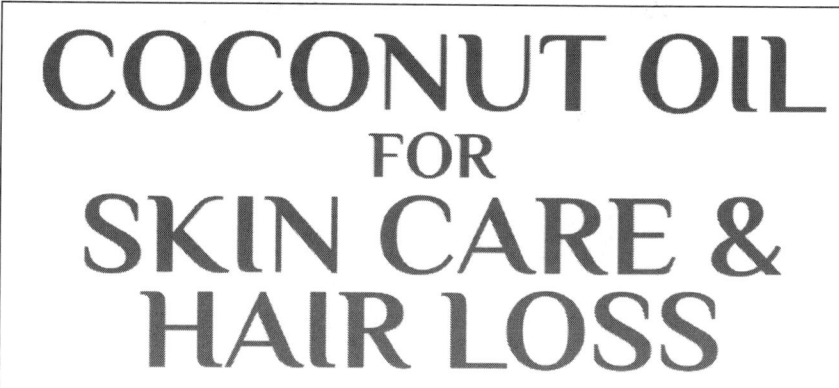

A Step By Step Guide For Using Virgin Coconut Oil For Youthful Skin And Healthy Hair

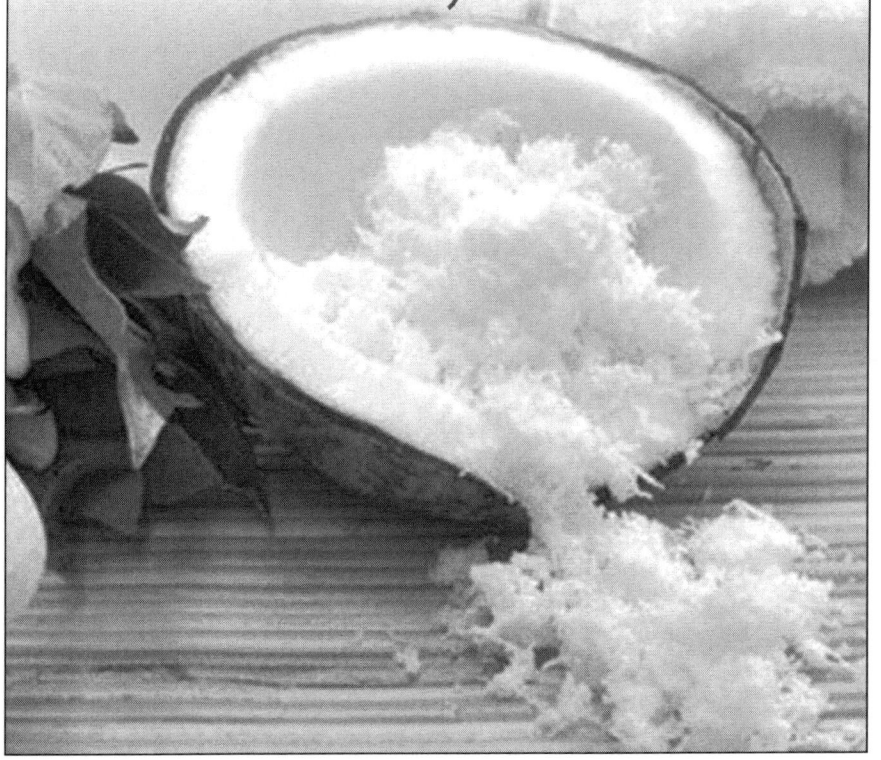

Copyright 2014 by Lindsey Pylarinos - All rights reserved.

In no way is it legal to reproduce, duplicate, or transmit any part of this document in either electronic means or in printed format. Recording of this publication is strictly prohibited and any storage of this document is not allowed unless with written permission from the publisher. All rights reserved.

COCONUT OIL FOR SKIN CARE & HAIR LOSS

Table Of Contents

Introduction 7

Chapter 1: A Brief History 9

Chapter 2: Kinds of Coconut Oil 12

Chapter 3: The Processes and Why It's Important for You to Know 16

Chapter 4: Coconut Oil for Skin Care 18

Chapter 5: Coconut Oil for Healthy Hair 20

Chapter 6: Other Beauty Tricks 23

Conclusion 25

Introduction

I want to thank you and congratulate you for purchasing the book, *Coconut Oil for Skin Care & Hair Loss*.

This book contains proven steps and strategies on how to use virgin coconut oil for youthful skin and healthy hair.

Coconut oil is commonly known as something edible; an important ingredient that plays a vital role to some of the food that tropical countries are very well familiar with. But since the supply of coconut oil has reached and developed in other parts of the world aside from the tropical ones, a great number of other uses have risen from the consciousness of the people.

Coconut oil has always been around you but it may have often gone unnoticed. Today, there are already innovated ways on how to make use of coconut oil, ways that are actually beneficial to your health. Aside from that, it can also serve as a beauty essential; one that you would want and need for healthy, beautiful skin and hair. In this book you will know how you can use coconut oil to your advantage.

The best thing about considering coconut oil as a beauty regimen is that it is a natural product, as if it is Mother Nature's own gift for you, in her desire to make you even more beautiful. With the kind of technology that human civilization has invented and developed, now there are various ways of attaining or maintaining beauty. There are chemicals that treat your hair to condition it the way you want it—soft, shiny, fragrant, and damage-free. There are also invented chemicals which are used to minimize the cells in your skin that cause darkening. Although these chemicals can be effective, they are not exactly safe. Some hair treatment can give you the hairstyle that you fancy but it can also cause hair loss and dryness. The same is also true for your skin; there are whitening products that make your skin vulnerable to the sun's rays which may lead to sickness due to the weakening of your skin's protective layer, so that in the process of being fairer you get exposed to the harm that the environment may cause upon your skin and your entire health.

Being beautiful doesn't have to mean being in danger, or having to risk your health for the sake of beauty. Coconut oil can give you soft, shiny, fragrant, and damage-free hair as well as fairer skin without putting your safety on the line. The fact that it is a natural product reduces the chances of danger that you could most likely get when you continue to use chemical-based beauty products.

Read on to find out how coconut oil can change your looks, and your life.

Thanks again for purchasing this book, I hope you enjoy it!

Chapter 1: A Brief History

According to recent studies, coconut oil is actually good for you. What most people might not know is that coconut oil has always been good for you, and that its culinary, medicinal, and cosmetic uses were not just recently discovered. The use of coconut oil in various occasions has been patronized since decades ago. But over the course of time, its image as a healthy treat was trampled by speculations of it being part of an unfit diet because of the amount of fat and cholesterol it contains. Going through coconut oil's brief history will shed some light on this subject.

Over the last three thousand nine hundred sixty years, coconut oil has always been used as a food product, but its potential for pharmaceutical purposes has also been discovered. The people of earlier times thought that growing coconut trees would be a good investment,and even the people of today would still agree; because although it might take a long time before it is ready to be harvested, the entirety of the tree is of good use for various situations and occasions. All of it was and still is good for harvesting—the bark and the strong wood can build the foundations of humble homes, the long and big leaves were used as roofs and plates, but the most promising part of the coconut tree was its fruit. The coconut itself had various uses—the coconut flesh, milk, water, and the coconut oil.

Centuries ago, during the time of richer nations' expeditions, European explorers found it fascinating how native people of the lands used coconut products to effectively rise from the state of their daily lives. It can be found in West Africa, the

Indian subcontinent, most Asian counties, as well as the Central and the South of America.

Coconut products have secured a place in history even before the manufacturers came into the picture. During the Second World War, the water that comes from coconuts was used as a substitute for saline solutions which saved many lives of injured soldiers. When the war had finally ended, coconut took on a different role. The Englishmen used it as margarine while the Americans turned it into butter.

Although it was a glorious time for coconut, there was a point in history that practically banned coconut oil along with other types of oils and fatty products. When studies conducted in the United States suggested that the primary causes for their adult citizens' short span of mortality are heart-related diseases due to the excessive consumption of fatty foods, coconut oil was one of the suspects for such a crime. Referred to as being part of a "Deadly Diet,"Americans ceased to patronize coconut products and favored polyunsaturated oils instead; failing to realize that coconut oil is pharmaceutically different from other natural oils. It is exactly the fatty acid that coconut oil contains which is responsible for the benefits that you can get out of using it as products that are known to men and women alike. Its fatty acids, like lauric acid for example, is actually one of the reasons why coconut oil has always been useful.

Many years later, in the time you know of as the present, the people is in need of a more affordable product that is just as effective; a product that would supplicate or at least act as a substitute or an alternative solution for the health demands of their daily lives. Today, coconut oil is able to aid the healing of and recovery from Alzheimer's disease, type 1 and

2 diabetes, and Candida infection. It has also been proven helpful in the process of weight loss, preserving muscle mass, and promoting ketosis.

After the negative campaign against deadly diets that practically ruined the reputation of coconut oil, it is back and it is on the rise to prove its worth not just in the market but also in the lives of different people, working its medicinal magic to promote a lifestyle lived with good health and wellness. It has alsoproven its progressive advancement in taste when it comes to food graced with generous amounts of coconut oil that you'll be dying to taste, and what just might be your next favorite beauty best friend.

Even until today, coconut oil is still performing miracles in the lives of people in the fields of food, medicine, and beauty.

Chapter 2: Kinds of Coconut Oil

There are two kinds of coconut oils to choose from and both have their own traits that may be beneficial for all. It is important to know the type of coconut oil that you are using so as to maximize its uses for you and avoid any unnecessary situations due to a lack of information. Debates have been going on from the beginning about which coconut oil is better, the refined or unrefined; but both have their fair share of contributions to the world.

Choosing which coconut oil to use can affect the results of what you are going to use it for. When cooking food, for instance, without prior knowledge you can commit the mistake of using unrefined coconut oil. Although it is edible too, nonetheless, it is still advisable to limit your cooking to refined coconut oil because it has already undergone a series of processes that thoroughly filtered it—making it safer and ideal when it comes to using coconut oil for the purpose of human consumption.

However, when it comes to purposes that involve beauty and pampering, a larger percentage of women prefer to use virgin coconut oil. Because virgin coconut oil is unrefined, it has only gone through a process which aims to make it hygienic without necessarily combining it with other chemicals. That way, its natural state would not have been entirely tampered with. According to the testimonials of women who have used it, this makes the unrefined coconut oil perfect for hair and skin treatments.

Deciding which brand that sells coconut oils is yet another thing. Since the product they sell can be used almost anywhere around your body, as will be tackled in this book later on, it is wise to know if the label you are putting on your body can be trusted—especially if you are planning to go with virgin coconut oil. The fact that it is unrefined should make you speculative as a consumer, about how the company or coconut farm processes their oils.

Both refined and unrefined coconut oils have their advantages and disadvantages, over other types of oils (organic or not), and over each other. The key to maximizing the full potential of both is research. Knowing the power of a certain product can also be of great help to your day-to-day activities. You can even combine coconut oil with other natural products to create something that you can use in innovating your daily beauty and hygiene routine. One good example is mixing coconut oil with brown sugar and vanilla. All three natural products can make a moisturizer that is better than the chemical-based lotion you usually spread across your body.

Refined Coconut Oil

One type of coconut oil is the refined variety. This type is perfect for those who enjoy deep frying foods. It is actually made from copra, which is the dried coconut. Once processed through a series of filtering its impurities to make it safe for consumption, it becomes the end product of refined, bleached, and deodorized (RBD) oil. Having been refined, this type of coconut oil is tasteless and does not contain the fragrance of coconut, but it is most commonly used for deep frying because this oil is able to withstand the high temperature.

Refined coconut oil is ideal for massive production or for cooking for a good number of people because it costs cheaper. Using refined coconut oil is also a great way to pamper yourself after a long day without having to spend so much salon service when you wish to stay on track of your budget. It is commonly used as a bath soap to moisturize the skin

Unrefined Coconut Oil

Another type is what is commonly known as the virgin coconut oil. This is famous in the market because of its effectiveness when it comes to beautification and being safe for the health. It is made from the first pressing of raw coconut which explains why the virgin coconut oil you can purchase in a grocery store still contains the fragrant smell of coconuts, as compared to the refined coconut oil which has already been deodorized.

Using the mechanical contraptions, the fresh coconut is processed without having to include any chemicals, which is how it got its name. The manner by which it was extracted can determine the strength of its flavor, but the basis for a well refined or virgin coconut oil is the mildness of its flavor and its scent.

One of the great things about virgin coconut oil is that it can last for up to two years without spoiling. This is credited to its high saturated fat content which makes the process of oxidation slower. Because of this, it becomes resistant to acquiring pungent odor and taste.

Unrefined coconut oil is expected to be more nutritious than refined coconut oil. Without being subjected to too much heat and additives, it is able to retain the nutrients that raw and pure coconuts possess. For this reasons, virgin coconut oils tend to be more expensive than the refined ones.

Chapter 3: The Processes and Why It's Important for You to Know

Coconut oil is known to provide medicinal and beauty essential alternatives that are safe and effective; but before it becomes such, it goes through processes that perfect its purpose in the everyday lives of men and women. There are two ways on how to extract coconut oils. One is the *dry process*. This process takes the meat out of the coconut and extracts it from the shell. Once it has been taken out of its shell, the coconut's meat is dried under the sun or in a fire. The dried extracts will later on turn it into copra which will be pressed with solvents, thus producing the coconut oil.

This process makes virgin coconut oil unsuitable for human consumption and therefore must be purified before including it in any food to prevent compromising health. Because the process involves exposing it in the open field while facing the sun for a couple of days or months until it is dried according to desired results, there are possibilities of insects stopping by on what is supposed to be edible. There are big chances of it getting dirt and dust while waiting for it to dry, and it isn't unlikely for field rodents to make an eventual visit as well. This makes it prone to fungal formation; this is also why it takes a long time to have it cleaned. When it is further extracted and purified, that is the only time when the oil used in cooking is finally produced.

The other way of extracting coconut oil is through the *wet process*. This makes use of the raw coconut instead of the dried copra. The difficulty in this process is recovering the oil after the breaking of emulsion. Boiling the oil from a long time can be the cause of this but it isn't advisable because it produces a discoloration in the oil itself.

There is also a process of *hydrogenation* wherein the oil is processed further to combine hydrogen with unsaturated fats to make it more saturated. The process of *fractionation* involves separating a fraction of the whole oil to be removed for specific purposes. For instance, a certain amount of acid from the whole coconut oil will be separated for the specific purpose of combining it with other chemicals for medicinal uses.

Because the primary topic of this book is about how coconut oil can help beautify your hair and skin in the form of shampoo and conditioner, lotion and moisturizer, it is important to know about the processes that the products go through. This will give you a background of the product that you are applying on your body. Being able to identify the kind of product that you use in your day-to-day life gives you the leverage of taking care of yourself better.

In choosing which coconut oil product to use, you must always take into consideration its contents aside from the coconut oil. Knowing what you might be allergic to is also prudent. Although natural products are safe by themselves, the processes they go through may have altered their composition and turned them into something that could be harmful for your health.

Wanting to have beautiful hair and flawless skin is not a crime. We are all entitled to a certain right to do what we must to feel confident and presentable, but never at the expense of our well-being.

Chapter 4: Coconut Oil for Skin Care

Coconut oil is used for a variety of purposes; one of them is for taking care of your skin. As mentioned in the conclusion of the previous chapter, it is crucial to be informed about the processes your product went through and the other chemicals that are mixed with it. You have to ask yourself how many of the chemicals listed on your products' container you would not want to be inside you. Everything you apply on the surface of your skin affects the layers beneath and even deeper; these include the toxins that can trigger skin diseases.

One solution is to find an alternative that you can trust. Using a product that is also edible is considered safer since you have it inside your body by way of consumption. Coconut oil is anti-bacterial. Taking that into perspective, you can see how coconut oil is helpful in controlling skin conditions that may be caused by germs and fungi. Unlike the usual skin whitening lotion you can buy at your local store, coconut oil is not greasy. With an ample amount spread generously throughout the body, you won't even get a sticky feeling at all. It's hard to feel that it's even there, except for your skin getting softer.

Some lotions, though fragrant, can cause skin rashes. Spreading coconut oil on your body not only gives your skin a lovely mild scent, but it also moisturizes it. Because coconut oil contains fats, it aids the wounds caused by acne and pimples on your skin to heal faster. It soothes your skin with its emollient properties, while repairing your skin's damaged tissues.

Coconut oil is also effective for achieving healthy, glowing skin. Its fatty acids nourish the skin to give you a revitalized complexion, making you look energized and blooming. It is also because of this reason that coconut oil can also hydrate the skin, protectingit from the damaging heat of the sun. Its properties also improve skin tone and prevent early wrinkling of the skin, making you look younger.

Most women's (including men's) facial dilemmas today include acne problems. Acne is a skin disease which is characterized by red scaly skin, blackheads, whiteheads, pimples, and pinheads. These are all cause by bacteria trapped in the pores. An effective way to get rid of these is through the help of coconut oil. The first thing you need to do is let your pores loose by facing a steam. The warmth of the steam will open your pores, giving way for the coconut oil to seep in. Apply coconut oil on your face and wipe after a minute, at least. Be mindful of the length of time you leave the oil on your face to avoid clogging your pores which may make things worse. Then simply wipe it away afterwards.

Coconut oil also contains antioxidants which relaxes your skin and eliminates dead skin cells to prevent your skin from flaking and dryness. And just when you think it's only good for the face, coconut oil is also discovered to be effective on the skin under your arms. It is a natural deodorant because it kills the bacteria that cause the bad odor in your armpits.

Chapter 5: Coconut Oil for Healthy Hair

What's In It for You?

As much as coconut oil is good for the skin, it also has a number of benefits for the hair. There are other natural products that have been used in shampoos and conditioners to treat the hair such as sunflower seeds, almond extracts, olive, minerals, and rose petals to name a few. But most of these can only do so much to coat the hair to protect it from being damaged, make it shiny, and soft.

Coconut oil is special in a way because it not just coats the hair strands but also penetrates the scalp and the hair strands' cortex. This means that by using coconut oil, your hair will not be confined to just being soft and shiny, but also strong with an improved flexibility. That having been said, it can be concluded that coconut oil makes your hair less prone to split ends and more protected from everyday damages caused by regular combing and styling.

Most oils just sit on the surface of your hair and are most likely to rinse off easily; but since coconut oil penetrates your hair, it doesn't sit on your hair's surface but repairs and protects it from the inside. Use it sparingly but spread generously especially on the tips of your hair for best results.

Everyone wants to grow healthy and beautiful hair, but that will not be possible if your hair is not growing properly in the first place. You might be surprised to know that your overall health actually affects the growth of your hair. It's important to know how the parts of your body are connected with each other. Making sure that your body takes in enough vitamins

COCONUT OIL FOR SKIN CARE & HAIR LOSS

to keep your health in check is also making sure that your beauty is maintained.

Many people are now using coconut oil to aid their hair's growth; with just the right amount and the proper application of coconut oil, you can have the hair you've always wanted by allowing your scalp to absorb the vitamins it needs for your hair to grow properly right from its roots.

One of coconut oil's basic components is lauric acid. This is a fatty acid which helps protect your hair by binding its proteins. Through this, hair strands are secured from the roots and will therefore not easily break. The protein binding property of coconut oils areproven to be more effective than sunflower oil and minerals, two of the most commonly used natural ingredients in a majority of shampoo and conditioning products.

Just as coconut oil moisturizes the skin, it also serves the same purpose for the hair. It conditions the hair from within, making it smoother. It is also a miracle worker for those whose eternal hair problems include dandruff and lice. The coconut oil's antifungal properties prevent these from growing in your hair.

Beautiful hair means healthy hair; coconut oil helps you achieve this by providing vitamins that are vital for your hair's beautiful and healthy growth. Coconut is rich in vitamin E, vitamin K and iron which are nutrients that maintain your hair's glow and softness.

Another great benefit that comes from using coconut oil on your hair is that improves your blood circulation. Next time you apply coconut oil on your hair, take time to massage your scalp. This provokes the stimulation of your blood circulation and gives the follicles of your hair the amount of oxygen it needs.

Starting Off

Now that you know the benefits of using coconut oil, you can now start your journey towards achieving and maintaining a healthier and more beautiful hair. You can either apply it on your hair before or after shampooing with your regular product. It is recommended for people with straight hair to apply coconut oil before shampooing while those with thicker curly hair are advised to apply it before and after their hair has been washed.

The first thing you have to do is apply an ample amount of coconut oil onto your scalp and massage gently to make sure that the oil is spread throughout your head. You have to allot at least thirty minutes for leaving your hair like this; an hour or so, for those with more hair problems, depending on the damage. After massaging your scalp, focus on your hair strands. You can wash it afterwards with your regular shampoo.

While you shampoo your hair with the coconut oil still there, you may notice how softer and smoother your hair has already gotten, although the results may vary after shampooing, depending on the type of hair you have. Note that our body's general health practices affect our hair's growth, this is why what might be an amazing result of using coconut oil for some, isn't so amazing for others. It's always best to take care of your overall health before problematizing beauty alternatives.

Chapter 6: Other Beauty Tricks

Aside from the already mentioned benefits of using coconut oil, there are still quite a number of ways by which you can use coconut oil for some beauty tricks. After a fun and long night out with your friends, you arrive home with your face sticky because of the mixture of make-up and the density of the atmosphere outside. You think washing your face would be enough and putting on some cold cream; but just because you can't see it, doesn't mean it isn't there. Coconut oil is a good make-up remover. There won't even be a hint of black line from your smudged mascara. Simply rub a small amount of coconut oil on your face, especially the eye area and gently wipe it away with a warm cloth after a few minutes. It is good to know that the skin of the eye area is actually thinner than the rest of your face. Wearing too much eye make-up can make the skin around your eyes age faster.

Another reason to love coconut oil is for the blessing it brings to unshaven legs. Thanks to the properties of coconut oil, you can have shaved soft and smooth legs without the need for a shaving cream. Before taking a bath, spread the coconut oil on your legs. Once in the shower, you can lather your legs with your regular soap and then shave it before rinsing. The smoothness that your legs will have is amazing.

For women with babies in the house, coconut oil can also be a good alternative for baby wipes. It can even prevent and heal diaper rash. To make your own homemade baby wipes, simply apply at least two teaspoons to your cotton or soft cloth and wipe gently on the baby's infected area.

Coconut oil also serves the purpose of toothpaste when

mixed with baking soda. You can also use it as a lip balm, personal lubricant, first aid, and sun burn relief by applying a small amount of oil on your dry areas in circular motion. It can cure a sore throat. It helps in healing stretch marks, psoriasis, dermatitis, and eczema; and many more.

If you're still unconvinced about the wonders that coconut oil has in store for you, you really have to check it for yourself because you are already missing out on a lot of beautiful possibilities.

Conclusion

Thank you again for downloading this book!

I hope this book was able to help you to realize the health and beauty benefits of using natural products and why you should really begin to consider adding coconut oil to your health and beauty essentials. There are a lot of other natural products that you can explore which are also good for both your physical well-being and gaining self-esteem by achieving your desired glow, but if you have only started to think it over, using coconut oil is a great way to introduce you to the rest of it.

I also hope that you have learned to value being healthy rather than merely being pretty. There are a lot of discovered and invented ways on how to achieve and maintain youth and beauty, but only a handful really offer safe, effective, and lasting results. Being a wise customer is important in ensuring that you get to buy the right product for your needs.

Your hair and your skin are two of the features that people notice first about you, so it's only fitting to see to it that they are well taken care of.

The next step is to try it for yourself. Coconut oil has a lot of potential uses for your everyday health and hygiene practices. Perhaps it's about time that you give it a try. But you must always remember that being beautiful doesn't mean having to sacrifice your health to attain it.

Finally, if you enjoyed this book, please take the time to share your thoughts and post a review on Amazon. We do our best to reach out to readers and provide the best value we can. Your positive review will help us achieve that. It'd be greatly appreciated!

Thank you and good luck!

Oil Pulling Therapy For Beginners:

BY LINDSEY PYLARINOS

Detoxify & Heal Your Mouth, Teeth, Gums & Body With Coconut Oil Through Natural Oil Pulling

Oil Pulling Therapy For Beginners

Detoxify & Heal Your Mouth, Teeth, Gums & Body With Coconut Oil Through Natural Oil Pulling

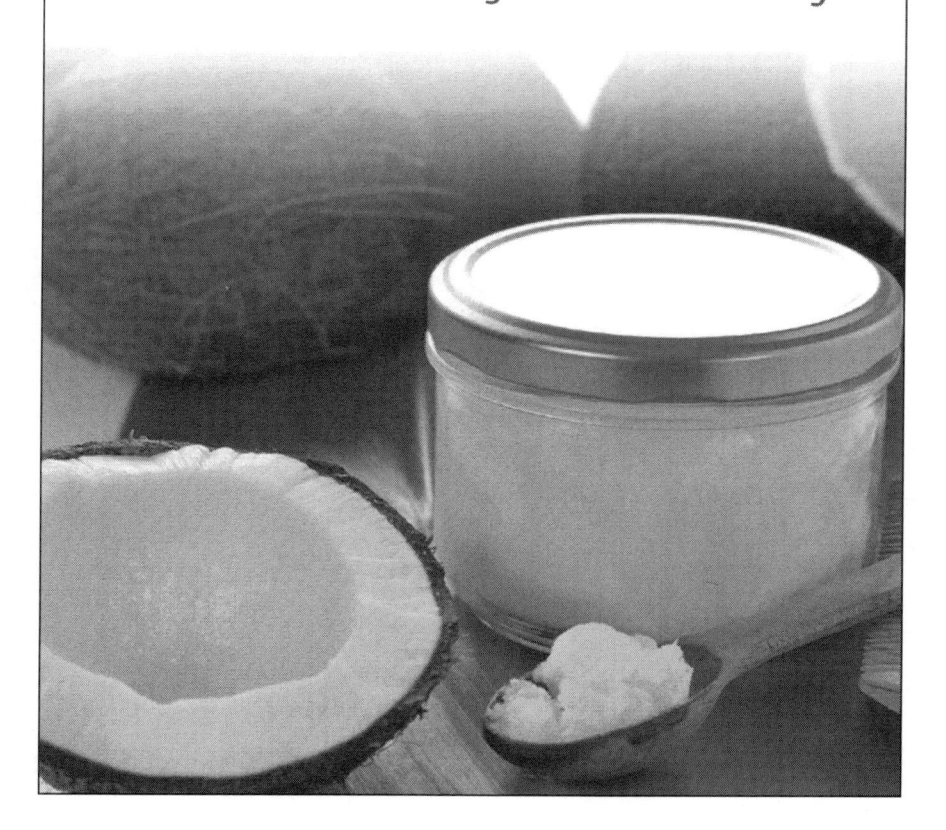

Copyright 2014 by Lindsey Pylarinos - All rights reserved.

In no way is it legal to reproduce, duplicate, or transmit any part of this document in either electronic means or in printed format. Recording of this publication is strictly prohibited and any storage of this document is not allowed unless with written permission from the publisher. All rights reserved.

Table of Contents

Introduction 33

Chapter 1 – The Oil Pulling Therapy "Health Craze" 34

Chapter 2 – So What Does Oil Pulling Really Do to You? ... 37

Chapter 3 – Because Oral Health Matters 40

Chapter 4 – Getting It On With the Oil Pulling Habit 44

Chapter 5 – More Oil Pulling Considerations 50

Conclusion 52

Introduction

I want to thank you and congratulate you for purchasing the book, Oil Pulling Therapy For Beginners: Detoxify & Heal Your Mouth, Teeth, Gums & Body With Coconut Oil Through Natural Oil Pulling.

This book contains proven steps and strategies on how to exploit the wonders of oil pulling not only for good oral health but also for our body's total health and wellbeing as well. Discover the secrets to be had and the great results that await you after reading this E-book.

Thanks again for purchasing this book, I hope you enjoy it!

Chapter 1 – The Oil Pulling Therapy "Health Craze"

What if you discover an ancient remedy that folks from all generations have used to improve their oral health and wellbeing, and at the same time have provided them with amazing detox benefits, and best of all, fix a whole lot of other medical problems? What if the best way to bring about all these benefits would be to simply swish oil all over your mouth for about 20 minutes everyday? Wouldn't you be intrigued? Would you not be interested? You should! This e-book will talk about the so-called "oil pulling" or "swishing" health craze and why it was a success story to people living in the past and in the present.

This ancient Ayurvedic remedy is designed for oral health, detoxification, and rejuvenation. It is actually a simple practice that presents quite remarkable results. Oil pulling involves using pure oils to effectively pull out fungus, bacteria, and other harmful organisms from the human mouth, gums, teeth, and all the way down to the throat. Many may have already heard of it, but they have yet to try it. One thing was made clear though, the oil pulling process has that exciting, mystical vibe surrounding it, which made many more eager and want to try it.

Oil pulling originated in India, appearing in the early Ayurvedic medicine texts (better known as traditional Indian medicine), and is highly considered these days as alternative medicine concepts known as Charaka Samhita. Here, you consume a tablespoonful of oil into your mouth during the mornings, and you pull or "swish" all around against your gums and teeth without ever swallowing it. Other sources recommend using sesame oil, as it is supposedly man's best friend, though others would be heard swearing by sunflower or coconut oil (others even warn against using coconut oil).

You are supposed to swish it all around for a good 20 minutes before spitting the oils out. And when it's out already, the clear and sparkling oil morphs into a whitey and milky-like substance full of the bacteria and toxins it had drawn out due to all that swishing. Sound's legit? Based on past experiences by generations in the past all the way to the present, it is legit. It works!

What Science Has to Say About the Oil Pulling Process and Sesame Oil

Scientific studies were quick and yet methodical to point out all the goodies to be had in the oil pulling process. The use of sesame oil here is critical; sesame oil, while it possesses a high concentration of polyunsaturated fatty acids and Vitamin E, is also high in sesamin, antioxidant sesamol, and sesamolin. Now what does all these mean? The antioxidants were found to be able to stop negative cholesterol forms from being absorbed into the liver. Specific scientific studies also revealed significant and helpful antibacterial capacities of the venerable sesame oil. The same studies highly support the oil pulling process when it comes to gingivitis and dental cavity prevention.

Another study conducted back in 2007 looked into the positive effects oil pulling using sunflower oil on cases of plaque and gingivitis on both soft and hard oral tissues. The results acknowledged that doing oil pulling for 45 days significantly reduces gingivitis.

In yet another 2008 study, it was discovered that the oil pulling process had remarkably reduced the total bacteria count within the mouth, which also proposed a marked reduction in dental cavity susceptibility overall. Here. The antibacterial properties of sesame oil was also put under the lens, and was found to have a positive effect on Streptococcus mutans, another disorder in the mouth.

All these studies painted a very clear picture on the ability of the oil pulling process to reduce bacteria significantly, from 10 to 35 percent. And after oil pulling for 40 days, it was discovered that oral bacterial afflicting the study participants were reduced down to 20%. Moreover, about half of the population of the study participants showed a significant reduction in the human body's susceptibility to dental caries.

Chapter 2 – So What Does Oil Pulling Really Do to You?

The oil pulling process (even if it focuses on the human mouth) literally heals every working part of your body, eventually making you fit and healthy in the long run. Nutritionists and functional medicine specialists have seen positive results. Although the oil pulling concept has already started to gain steam in the Western World in recent years, dental professionals are still confused when it comes to proper responses to patient cases who have already adopted this particular alternative therapy. The thing is the longer you do the swishing of oil into your mouth (specifically the teeth and gums), the more microbes will be dug and taken away. You have to swish the oil enough until it turns into milky white. When this happens you can be certain that harmful bacteria has been removed.

Using coconut oil for the process works excellently for teeth whitening. And at the same time, it is valued for its anti bacterial/viral properties, which means it could help us detox our body, deal with annoying sinuses, and strengthens the teeth and gums as well. Where we are going to see that it would not work is when an individual is not currently addressing gastrointestinal issues, and is also bloated from intestinal parasites, an imbalance of good bacteria, and candida overgrowth. Oil pulling basically works effectively. The best part of it all is that it doesn't end there. There's so much that we could still discover, so much that the oil pulling process could do for our personal health.

Yet here we are, enjoying all its known benefits, which is the following:

- It whitens the teeth,
- It strengthens the gums, teeth and jaw overall. The process is very helpful in cases of sensitive teeth. It was even reported to have aided TMJ sufferers,
- It prevents cavities and gingivitis from forming up,
- It helps us deal with our acne problems, including psoriasis, eczema, and other persisting skin care issues,
- And as already mentioned before, it helps in your general detox efforts, which is very important to overall health in the long run,
- If you are a party animal and you like to drink much, oil pulling is good news because it can cure your hangovers (and even migraines) with ease,
- The oil pulling practice helps you manage your sleep issues,
- It helps clear out the sinuses and aid allergy sufferers in general,
- If you are suffering from halitosis, oil pulling helps freshen up your breath by getting rid of common oral problems,
- Oil pulling helps you to solve your general pain issues,
- It helps prevent lips, mouth, and throat dryness,
- Reduces arthritis inflammations,
- Help support normal kidney functions,
- The oil pulling process is also a possible holistic TMJ treatment, including the soreness in your jaws.
- It also helps you to manage any weird hormonal imbalances, and
- The list goes on.

From a mechanical perspective, everything would start to make sense. Now we all know that tooth decay is primarily the result of bacteria thriving all over your mouth, but with this simplified oral health technique, chances are you will have an improved dental health. And everyone believed that total health and wellbeing starts with good oral health.

Beyond the Mouth

Health practitioners of this ancient Ayurvedic concept firmly believed that the oil pulling process could affect well beyond the throat and mouth. In fact, many of today's holistic practitioners are pretty confident about oil pulling for various common health concerns.

Based on studies and past experiences, it is widely believed that the oils used in the process aid the human body's lymphatic system as significant harmful bacteria are taken out to give space for beneficial microflora to flourish in a new healthy environment instead. And because of such holistic perspective, the oil pulling process is also brought to bear as a preventative health practice for other common health conditions.

Some experts believe that the miraculous nature of oil pulling can be translated into a speedy cure and recovery of certain acute disease in just as little as 2 to 4 days. Other chronic diseases on the other hand would require more time for the oil pulling process to do its trick – sometime to a year. You only need to be persistent in your efforts and drive to improve your health for the better.

Chapter 3 – Because Oral Health Matters

The thing is, oil pulling is never magic, but rather your mouth is. At the least part of it, when you have a healthy mouth, or when it is working properly, your mouth is actually your gateway to overall health. The oil pulling process is just among ways to clean up your mouth with efficiency so your body could concentrate on other areas that needs addressing.

In a nutshell, the oil pulling process creates friction that can be characterized as like having a soap-like function that cleans up the mouth. It does not really matter what oil type will be used in the process, and sesame oil is cheap and readily available to regions in the world where folks have been using oil pulling for a long time now. Either way, oil pulling is a great way of addressing gingivitis. The reason for this is that the process reduces the bacteria thriving in the mouth – it reduces the strep mutans bacteria present in saliva and plaque that causes cavities.

However, you must understand that the oil could only penetrate a millimeter deep. The more serious infections would most likely be 3 to 5 millimeters deeper. This means oil pulling will not really be helpful to those already suffering from gum disease. If they insist, they could end up losing their teeth instead.

What this chapter hopes to achieve however, is to answer, from a health and nutritional standpoint, if oil pulling is that big fix for almost all that we have been complaining about our body. And yes it is the big fix! As already agreed upon by various experts, a dramatic improvement in an individual's oral health positively affects everything. Whenever we make a serious effort to improve our oral health, we inadvertently improve other health issues in our body.

The connection is very strong. How so? Individuals suffering from bad oral hygiene are always at risk to various cardiovascular issues like stroke and heart attack, including risks to pneumonia as well. Men suffering from periodontal disease are in danger of developing erectile dysfunction. The same case also applies to diabetes. An improved oral health could do so much to help control different problems in diabetic patients. Pregnant women suffering from gum disease were also reported to give birth to lower birth-weight babies.

As you can see from all the situations cited, everything is connected. Good oral health affects everything. During post-oil swishing, patients can then enjoy skin clarity, improved sinuses, and decimated cavities.

For starters, your mouth is connected to you your sinuses and ear canal. If you achieve an improved oral hygiene via oil pulling, you can also expect a decreased ear and sinus infection. Your tooth infections may also be related to your sinus infections, though medical experts have discovered how improvement is achieved through Xylitol, a sugar substitute. Toothpastes containing Xylitol are also known to help decrease ear infections in kids down a good 50%.

What this tells us is that in our rush to give the oil pulling process a thumbs-up for its cure-all capabilities, what we have stumbled into instead is an old and proven way to clean the mouth more thoroughly and effectively at the same time than we would have known by now. And it would probably seem really appealing as "the new hit," instead of having to settle with our toothbrush and floss. But to do just that would definitely make you feel better as well. It's a proven oral health practice that will never go away.

If you have a healthier mouth, expect less inflammation within your body. You'll also feel fresh and in better moods for most part of the day. If you have a fresh mouth, you'll be confident talking to anyone you meet. It does so much to improve your self-esteem. You'll also be presented with more energy, as the presence of the gum disease infection keeps your body constantly dealing with this particular bacteria just to keep it away from your body and wreaking havoc. And this can be stressful to us. Once the chronic infections of the mouth improve, we both feel and look better then.

So swish away, because you are doing you whole body and wellbeing a great service, and besides you have an obligation to give your mouth the full attention it deserves. Oil pulling may not really address your cavities since they are virtually just out of reach, but the process targets those cavity-causing bacteria in the mouth instead, which is already effective on its own.

It's important not to forget the caveats here – you are not supposed to swallow the oil. There were some reported cases where the oil used was swallowed by accident, resulting to the lungs getting loaded with toxin particles, which then leads to the sufferers aspirating the dirty oil, and even developing pneumonia as well.

It is also worth noting that oil pulling should not be considered a substitute for brushing the teeth altogether, as others have suggested. Dental experts anywhere could be heard recommending the oral irrigator as an ideal cleaner to get into spaces in between teeth, and for preventing inflammation as well. There are some reported cases where patients still complain about inflammations in between their teeth even while doing oil pulling, though these are isolated cases only. This would suggest that oral irrigation and flossing still remains ideal.

When it comes to the case of mouthwashes however (not all of it though), oil pulling is highly regarded as a better substitute.

Chapter 4 – Getting It On With the Oil Pulling Habit

You can start oil pulling by putting a tablespoon of organic sesame oil (cold-pressed) into your mouth and then swishing it around for about 10-15 minutes before spitting it all out (imagine how you would do it with your mouthwash). After introducing the oil into your mouth, you can start pushing, swirling, and pulling it in between your teeth and all over your gums. You must let the oil brush through every part and corner of your mouth, except the throat of course. As already mentioned earlier, swallowing the oils used accidentally can be very bad, you wouldn't want to swallow the toxins, would you? It is also in your best interest not to let the oil get into contact with the throat since the swished oil is now carrying those removed toxic materials from the mouth. And absolutely no gargling as well!

In other cases, other oils are also used, such as sunflower oil, olive oil, and extra virgin cold-pressed coconut oil, although many consider sesame oil as the best oil to use for the oil pulling process. It is also recommended that you alternate using oils every after a couple of days to achieve the full effect of the process. Utilizing high quality organic oils is ideal for producing that multi-effect outcome many have craved for.

What happens is that the oils first mix with your saliva until it becomes white and thin-like. The lipids within the oils then begin to pull out the toxins settling on your saliva. As the oil swishes all over your mouth, tongue, teeth, and gums, it will continue absorbing the toxins until it becomes white, thick and viscous. And once it has reached such consistency, you have to spit them out before you accidentally reabsorb the toxins.

Oil pullers traditionally favor the virgin sesame oil. Some of them however, pointed out how they prefer raw coconut oil instead because of its anti-inflammatory, antibacterial, and even enzymatic properties that is presented to you in a package deal. You just swish the oils through and it will do the rest. This also provides you with an added benefit of ridding unwanted bacteria that your regular toothbrush would be having a hard time dealing with.

Aside from attracting and removing bacteria, parasites, and toxins that thrive in both your mouth and lymph systems, the swishing also pulls out mucus congestions that had settled down your throat, thus loosening up your sinuses at the same time. And this is a very amazing feat. With the aid of your saliva, such scary, unwanted undesirables would then bind with the oil you used. The pulling process also helps to strengthen the gums and teeth foundations by cleaning such areas thoroughly, and re-mineralize your teeth at the same time.

Spitting the Oils Out

It is important that once you are finished, you must spit the oils out into the toilet or trash, but never into the sink. The oil could easily solidify, eventually clogging the drain. You can then rinse your mouth using clean water 2 to 3 times. Drink a glass of water afterwards and relax. This is where you get that freshness and rejuvenation feeling.

wish

 an do the swishing at any time of the day, the perform the routine (especially if you are aiming for a more thorough detox) is in the mornings before having breakfast, or even before drinking your first glass of water for the day. One sensible reason to do this one is that you can easily integrate it to the rest of your morning routine. If you find it difficult to fit the process into your routine, you need not worry. Try to be creative. If you find it convenient to oil pull while in the shower, then by all means go ahead. This way, you would not be counting the minutes passing by hoping for it end so you could spit the oil out already.

The ancient Ayurveda healing concept encourages oil pulling in the mornings just right after cleaning the teeth and tongue, and when the stomach is still empty. You may do it an hour after drinking coffee, tea, water, or other liquids, but ideally not before breakfast. To add, the best time to pull would also be when you are not actually feeling well.

Recommended oil pulling frequency is placed at 3 times a day just to enhance this healing process (ideally before meals), though it all depends on you.

The oil pulling process is also known to increase mouth saponification – this creates a soapy environment that function to cleanse the mouth. This is made possible due to the presence of the vegetable fat, which is considered an emulsifier in nature. What's more interesting is the oil's ability to weed out harmful bacteria and reduce fungal growth at the same time. Such oils are also able to aid the cellular restructuring process, as they are related to the lymph node functions, and including that of other internal organs.

The Effort Involved and Jaw Pain

Does the whole process require effort? Should the swishing of the oil all over the mouth be that hard? In most cases, individuals who gave it a try and documented their experience online complained how their jaws got a little bit crampy immediately while doing the swishing. Some could still remember how they were a little nauseous (which is normally acceptable since they just started the process), though advocates were strong to point out that you'll eventually get used to the swishing. And besides, should the cramping of your jaws persist, it could well be that you are swishing so fast that your jaws are pressured at all sides.

To better understand it, jaw pain is a common thing as you start your oil pulling routine for the first time. This is mainly because you are exerting effort and pressure into your jaw muscles and joints, which in most cases are not used very often. The oil pulling process, however, can strengthen your jaws (even to those with TMJ issues) if you try to build up gradually. It is also important that you do not overdo it as well.

As in most homeopathic medicinal styles, oil pulling should be a more relaxing process; it would not be wise to develop that "over speeding" habit like someone mad in his quest for instant results. The thing is, relax when you swish. Forget the discomfort. It's all in the mind.

Have fun with your oil swishing instead. This should help you manage the discomforts. Try humming a little song and getting into a rhythm while doing the swishing. You could also do some deep breathing sets through your nose. Condition your mind on how to enjoy this cleansing feeling, including the relaxation that comes from the absence of talking. Know that there's nothing quite like feeling fresh and light afterwards. Know that what you are doing is just right and healthy. And before you know it, you are already done with your swishing session for the day.

You also need to be consistent with your oil pulling. Experts highly recommend that an adequate swishing session would last for 20 minutes for each day. While this may seem too much to you now, take comfort in the fact that some folks get the job done in just 15 minutes, and some others reporting that they got results with just 10 minute-a-day oil swishing. Are you supposed to do this everyday? Experts are content doing oil pulling 5 times in a week.

If it so happens that you are allergic to particular oil types, you could simply make a switch to another oil type.

Another popular reason why people these days turn to oil pulling is the relief they get from their sinus and throat congestion problems. To point the obvious, the pace with which this takes effect is unbelievable. There are lots of cases where immediately after rinsing, pullers found out their throats have cleared and that they could blow their noses clearly. These pullers were also struggling with chronic sinus congestion problems, and it was a great relief having to swish oil everyday for 20 minutes. They claimed that their conditions greatly improved afterwards.

There are also those who started oil pulling to help improve their extremely sensitive gums and teeth. They gained favourable results in return as their gums have strengthened up and their teeth became whiter and livelier than before. And it didn't stop there, as the effect of the process also extended out to their skin, dramatically improving the life and texture.

Gagging Issues

When it comes to gagging, many users resort to es: in an effort to get used to the process and not to g
it. Before swallowing, they smell the oil in the spoon first to help condition them up for the swishing that would follow. Another effective way would be to avoid taking in solid coconut oil (that is if your using one). Take it only in its room temp state.

The opposite could work for others; they would rather take coconut oil in its solid state and then letting it melt inside their mouths.

Gagging is a common issue for many; experts believe the best way to combat it would be using oils with scents you are comfortable with. You could basically wipe some essential oils and raw unrefined coconut oil right under your nose just to get a good sense of it before you start swishing. If it so happens that you gag due to that oil feeling, you could add a couple of squirts of either pure or alkaline water, rose water, colloidal silver, or 3% food-grade peroxide to the oil that you'll use for your swishing. This would thin the oil down a bit just enough to make it tolerable and that you won't gag anymore.

Chapter 5 – More Oil Pulling Considerations

In the Case of Fillings

Many experts believe that oil pulling should be encouraged. This comes into light based on experiences of others who have fillings and were plagued mercury and other gases that becomes toxic inside the mouth, thus giving them headaches. One good reason for doing an oil pull would be the eradication of the toxins that have already accumulated on your mouth. And the fact that you spit the oil out carrying with it all the toxins removed from the process means the toxins are not detoxified through your body, which means so much to overall body health and wellbeing.

Another logical reason we need to consider here is how unfortunate it would be if those who have fillings cannot have access to the oil pulling process. And we all know most of us have fillings on our own.

In the Case Of False Teeth

Those with false teeth could also engage in oil pulling to keep their gums healthy at all times. The swishing of the oil should help prevent sores from happening due to false teeth structures that regularly come into contact with the gums as soon as they are planted and replanted in. The pulling also aids in addressing bad breath and detox issues as well.

A Good Combo to Try

Some experts have been hailing oil pulling together with the activated charcoal component as a great combo to better enhance the capabilities and benefits that we get from the process itself. Adding activated charcoal to your oil pulling routine using raw coconut oil is a great discovery. Not only does the combination pull the toxins on the mouth out of the body, prevent plaque, whitens teeth, and heal various gum issues, it does it faster more efficiently, and with less risks to detoxification side effects. You must be warned though, its not ideal that you do the oil pulling and activated charcoal combo routine if you are about to go out of the house or work as your tongue initially turns into a blackish gray due to the charcoal component. If you must, try brushing your tongue first. You can also try brushing your teeth using baking soda or DIY toothpastes. Rinse afterwards and you'll get amazing results.

Those using this particular combo also found it easier to put that tablespoonful of oil into their mouth. As the coconut oil melts on the spoon, add a 1/8 of a teaspoon of activated charcoal powder before swallowing and swishing it. And while at it, you could add 2 squirts of colloidal silver into your mouth. If you happen to have mercury fillings/amalgams or root canals, the introduction of activated charcoal prove to be an excellent way to reach out further and grab more toxins so they are spit out.

This should discourage what oil pulling using coconut oil could do to clean your mouth and body though. Pulling using coconut oil and spitting it out after 20 minutes rids you of your toxin accumulation problem. Adding activated charcoal simply takes your oil pulling routine to a whole new level.

Conclusion

Thank you again for purchasing this book!

I hope this book was able to help you to understand how there is so much hope for your oral health woes thru oil pulling.

The next step is to check out my other books.

Finally, if you enjoyed this book, please take the time to share your thoughts and post a review on Amazon. We do our best to reach out to readers and provide the best value we can. Your positive review will help us achieve that. It'd be greatly appreciated!

Thank you and good luck!

Healing Babies and Children with Aromatherapy for Beginners

BY LINDSEY PYLARINOS

Proven Steps on How to Use Essential Oils and Aromatherapy to Care for Babies and Children

Healing Babies & Children With Aromatherapy For Beginners

Proven Steps On How To Use Essential Oils & Aromatherapy To Care For & Heal Babies & Children

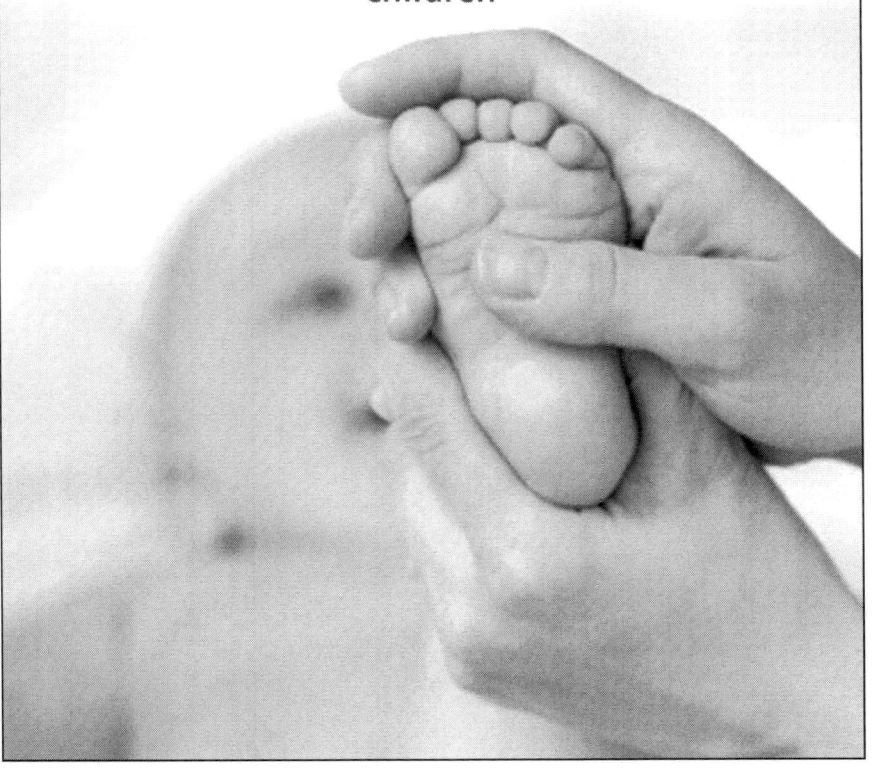

Copyright 2014 by Lindsey Pylarinos - All rights reserved.

In no way is it legal to reproduce, duplicate, or transmit any part of this document in either electronic means or in printed format. Recording of this publication is strictly prohibited and any storage of this document is not allowed unless with written permission from the publisher. All rights reserved.

Table of Contents

Introduction 59

Chapter 1: Introducing Babies to Aromatherapy 60

Chapter 2: Baby Massage Oils 63

Chapter 3: Essential Oils for Bath Time 66

Chapter 4: Essential Oils for Skin Healing 68

Chapter 5: Essential Oils for Inhalation and Room Diffusion 71

Chapter 6: Essential Oils for Tantrums 75

Chapter 7: Essential Oils for Coughs, Colds and Flu 77

Chapter 8: Essential Oils for Other Ailments and Health Purposes 81

Conclusion 84

Preview Of My Books 85

Introduction

I want to thank you and congratulate you for purchasing the book, *"Healing Babies and Children with Aromatherapy for Beginners: Proven Steps on How to Use Essential Oils and Aromatherapy to Care for Babies and Children"*.

This book contains proven steps and strategies on how to make use of Aromatherapy to better care for babies and children. Aromatherapy and using essential oils are both effective ways of making a child's life better. It's always good to help them become exposed to the great benefits that Aromatherapy can give early on as it will help them become healthier and more relaxed.

With the help of this book, you will learn how to introduce your children—babies included—to Aromatherapy and Essential Oils, how to use them for different situations, and how to create different types of oils for Aromatherapy.

Start reading this book now and turn your child's life for the better.

Thanks again for purchasing this book, I hope you enjoy it!

Chapter 1: Introducing Babies to Aromatherapy

Babies' skin is often sensitive and that's why you have to be careful with what you apply to them. And since you are going to make use of essential oils, you need not worry much because these oils come from natural sources which mean that they are safe to use.

However, since you are dealing with babies here, it would still be important to keep in mind some tips, such as:

- Do not use essential oils for babies younger than 3 months old. During this stage, babies are extremely sensitive and it would still be best to check with your doctor first before applying anything on them. Lavender and Chamomile are the first two oils that you can use for babies. Don't use eucalyptus oil unless babies are over 2 years of age as this may be too extreme for them.

- Dilute the oils with water well before using so that the oils will not be too strong for the babies.

- Do not give them essential oils orally!

- You don't have to be an expert when it comes to massaging babies or children—you only have to be very gentle and make sure that with each touch come love and affection. It's very important for a child to feel loved and wanted and that's what he/she should feel when you massage him/her with essential oils.

- 1% dilution or 5 drops essential oil to 2 Tbsp carrier oil is good for babies up to 2 years of age. After which, you can use 2% dilution or 10 drops essential oil per 2 Tbsp carrier oil already.

- And, you also have to make sure that you use only pure, essential oils. Synthetic oils and overly fragrant oils have no healing properties and won't make your babies/children feel better.

Here is a list of essential oils that you can use for babies less than 2 years of age:

- Chamomile
- Lavender
- Neroli
- Sweet Orange
- Mandarin
- Geranium
- Dill
- Tea Tree
- Rose
- Olive
- Sweet Almond
- Coconut

Essential Oils for Children over 2 years of age:

- Tangerine

- Rosemary

- Lemon

- Ginger (make sure to use only 1/3 of this though, or not as much as you use other oils as it is still quite "heavy" for kids)

You can use other kinds of oils once they are 3 years old and above. You may also mix other types of oils with what's written here as long as you do not use too much of them. Now, it's time to start making your own therapeutic oils that you can use for the kids.

Chapter 2: Baby Massage Oils

Giving your children the gift of time is still the best gift you can give. And, what better way to show your kids that you have time for them than by giving them a warm, genuine massage? Not only will you be able to apply essential oils on them, they'll also feel better because they'd know that their parent is willing to spend time with them and help them become better, healthier individuals, too!

Other reasons why it is important to give your babies/children a massage:

- A massage is able to stimulate one's nervous system;

- A massage is a great form of bonding with your child;

- A massage is actually able to improve digestion and blood flow, which are very important in living a healthy life;

- A massage helps clear the skin and helps in making it soft and supple and really nice to touch;

- A massage is a great way of detoxification as it helps clean the body and rid it of stress;

- And most importantly, it stimulates not just one's body but also one's brain, making way for holistic healing and truly healthy living.

Try these essential oil recipes below that are perfect for massaging your babies:

Daily Baby Massage Oil

Ingredients:

- 1 drop geranium
- 1 drop roman chamomile
- 1 drop lavender
- 30 ml sweet almond oil

Procedure:

- Blend all ingredients together and store in a glass bottle. You may use this daily.

Sleep Well, Little Child

Ingredients:

- ½ tsp olive oil
- 1 Tbsp apricot kernel oil
- 5 to 10 drops lavender essential oil
- ½ Tbsp coconut oil

Procedure:

- Pour all ingredients in a bowl and mix together before pouring in a glass bottle. This is best for babies 2 years and older.

Skin Healing Massage Oil

Ingredients:

- 2 Tbsp chamomile flowers
- 2 Tbsp calendula flowers
- 1 cup organic olive oil

Procedure:

- Heat water over medium heat then melt oil in a double boiler or glass bowl on water.

- Add chamomile and calendula flowers then just let heat stay at low or medium and wait until the oil becomes yellow and smells of calendula and chamomile already. Check water level so you can be sure that it has not evaporated or has not gotten overly hot.

- **Strain the flowers out then pour mixture in a glass bottle after cooling. Use as regular baby oil for massage.**

Chapter 3: Essential Oils for Bath Time

Children and babies appreciate it when they know that their bath water smells good. It lures them to love bathing and would help you to not have a hard time getting the babies cleaned and when it comes to taking care of them better. Plus, you'll certainly appreciate how great their bath water smells, too—it will help you relax and be soothed, as well.

Lavender and Chamomile Bath

Just add a single drop of chamomile or lavender to at least 20 ml water or full-fat milk and your baby will surely love bath time! This will also help the baby become less cranky and will help him sleep better after the bath. Using 1 to 3 drops of these essential oils per bath water would also be good.

Frankincense and Clary Sage

The mixture of Clary Sage and Frankincense is great because they are both naturally rejuvenating and soothing and can also relieve and relax tired muscles—which mean that you can use them for yourself, too.

Other Essential Oils that are meant for bath time:

- Bergamot
- Basil
- Rose
- Sandalwood

- Ylang-Ylang
- Juniper
- Marjoram (Marjoram is also great against insomnia and for baths that you'll let your baby take before bedtime)
- Cypress
- Eucalyptus
- Lemongrass
- Lemon
- Peppermint
- Fennel
- Rosemary
- Thyme

One or two drops of each oil is already good to keep the bath water fresh and great for your child. You may also use vegetable oil as the carrier base or pour the essential oils in milk to help soften your child's skin.

Chapter 4: Essential Oils for Skin Healing

Some babies may develop rashes or skin irritations. Eczema is very common among babies who have dry or sensitive skin. You'd know that your baby has eczema if there are red and itchy rashes on his/her skin.

With the help of doctor's prescriptions and with the essential oils listed below, you can be sure that your baby will be rid of all the bad stuff that he/she is experiencing when it comes to his/her skin. Also, with the use of essential oils, you can now avoid using steroid lotions or topical steroids which aren't really made from natural products and may cause some side-effects in the future.

Essential Oils to heal the skin:

(Just mix 1 to 5 drops of these oils with water and olive oil, as its base, and pour in a glass bottle for safety and storage. Using olive oil as base is important because it is also used in most creams, lotions and cures for skin irritation that you can find in the market and it is also a natural skin moisturizer. For babies 2 years and above, you can use 10 drops of these oils. Spread or massage on baby's skin thoroughly. You may also add these oils to Aloe Vera Gel as it makes skin healing even better and faster.)

A great recipe would be: 10 to 20 drops essential oil per 1 oz sunflower, olive or almond oil. Just choose from any of the essential oils below, or use 2 or 3 of them together with the vegetable oil base:

- **Chamomile Oil**—is great against inflammation and is also a good antiseptic.

- **Evening Primrose Oil**—is meant to treat eczema, especially for babies.

- **Calendula Oil**—is also great against inflammation and is popular for its tissue-healing and regeneration properties. It's important for babies to regenerate cells and tissues so that their skin will be more intact and supple.

- **Jasmine Oil**—Jasmine is known for its natural calming and soothing properties and that's why it always works to clear the skin.

- **Lavender Oil**—is a natural anti-septic and is very effective against inflammation. It is also a natural disinfectant and smells really relaxing and calming, too.

- **Tea Tree Oil**—this is great against mosquito or insect bites especially if you are travelling with your child to faraway places. It eases swelling and is also effective against inflammation plus you can be sure that your child will no longer feel pain or will no longer be itchy once tea tree oil is used.

Other Choices that have the same properties as oils mentioned above:

For dry skin:

- Sandalwood
- Rosewood
- Roman Chamomile

- Grapefruit
- Frankincense

For Oily/Sensitive Skin:

- Tea Tree
- Bergamot
- Lavender
- Manuka
- Myrrh
- Helichrysum
- Rosemary
- Geranium
- Blue Tansy

Make use of these essential oils and your baby's skin shall be soft and beautiful at all times—not to mention, you'll be able to get rid of his/her skin irritation/eczema, too!

Chapter 5: Essential Oils for Inhalation and Room Diffusion

An effective way of using aromatherapy to make sure that your baby is comfortable and healthy is by room diffusion. This way, you can be sure that your child will be able to inhale the scent of essential oils and be able to sleep better. There are different ways of doing this and these are:

Natural Room Freshener

You can do this by placing a bowl of water in the room, away from baby's head and from where it could drip or fall down and pouring a pint of water in. Add a drop of essential oil (Lavender is always a favorite) and just wait for the scent to steam or go around the room. The scent will now be well-circulated. You may use Roman Chamomile or Jasmine if the baby is not sleeping well. These will help him/her feel relaxed and ready to rest. Mandarin essential oil is also good in curing insomnia and in helping your baby sleep better—it'll help you sleep better, as well.

Scenting a Hanky

Another good way of using aromatherapy to keep your baby relaxed is by putting a few drops of lavender on a handkerchief and placing it near the baby who is sleeping. You may also place this on your shoulder while you are feeding the baby so that he/she will be able to associate the smell with security and comfort, and with feeling loved and taken care of, as well. Some other essential oil choices for pouring on a handkerchief include:

Jasmine, which is naturally calming and is said to help babies and even adults to easily fall asleep;

- Chamomile, a very relaxing oil that is best for almost all incidents and is definitely safe and gentle for babies;
- Rose, which is fragrant and calming in the best possible way.

A remedy for Insomnia

When your child is having a hard time getting to sleep, surely you'll have a hard time going to sleep, too. It's never nice having to deal with endless crying fits especially if you have no idea why your child finds it hard to sleep. It would be good to ask your doctor about this but if Insomnia really is the case, then you can try making use of essential oils to help your baby be able to sleep easily and also to give you some peace of mind. You can try mixing 3 drops ylang-ylang, 30 ml lime blossom oil, 3 drops noble chamomile, 20 ml sunflower oil and 2 drops Marjoram sweet and placing the mixture in a diffuser so your child will easily be able to inhale it. This way, he/she will easily be soothed and easily be able to fall asleep.

Scenting Children's Drawers

You may also use essential oils to ensure that your children's drawers or cabinets smell good and would help them feel relaxed instead of worried or panicky. You can do this by applying Chamomile or Lavender essential oils to cotton balls then placing them on the drawers, the way you would with moth balls. This is in fact better and more fragrant and relaxing than moth balls and are definitely safer for children, too. Plus, it'll help the drawers stay clean so you can be sure that your children only wear clothes that are clean, fragrant and comfortable.

As Cleansers for your child's bags and things

For older children, you may make use of essential oils to ensure that their things are not only clean but will also help them feel better and secure. You can do this by adding a few drops of Mandarin, Lemon, Orange or Bergamot Oil with water then moistening a clean cloth with the mixture and using it to clean your child's belongings.

For inhalation

You can use essential oils to help your children breathe better. Airways can be cleared by inhaling some essential oils. However, it is not recommended for children with asthma or for those who are having an asthma attack at the moment. To do this, just place 1 to 8 drops of essential oil in a clean, dry cloth and use the cloth to inhale the oils. Orange, Mandarin, Lavender, Chamomile and Jasmine are all good choices that will help your child breathe better.

You may also try mixing a drop of ginger, a drop of bergamot and a drop of sweet orange and putting them in a tissue for inhalation purposes.

Use a Diffuser

You may also use a ready-made diffuser that you can buy from the market. Make sure that you do not place it really near the baby, though. Just add a drop of the essential oil of your choice to a tablespoon of water and place it in the diffuser and turn it on. Your baby's room will definitely smell better and be a relaxing place because of this.

With the tips mentioned above, your child will surely be calmed and relaxed in no time—and you will, too.

Chapter 6: Essential Oils for Tantrums

It's very normal for babies to act out or have tantrums, at times. But of course, tantrums are not very nice and easy things to deal with especially if you have no idea how to deal with them. Tantrums are big tests of one's patience and will definitely get you thinking how you can manage taking care of your children and feeling like you have to deal with the tantrums. Lucky for you, there are some essential oils that you can use to ease your child's tantrums and to also help you feel calm. Here are some of the oils that you can try and what you should do with them:

- **Lavender**—Just pour 1 drop of Lavender oil on your shoulder or on a cloth then place it on your shoulder while rocking the baby and the baby will surely be able to sleep easily. Mixing Lavender with Mandarin Oil is also great in putting your baby to sleep.

- **Sweet Orange**—also known as the oil of happiness, Sweet Orange is very effective against tantrums and in helping babies feel happy and relaxed. You can just place a drop or two of this in a diffuser so your baby would be able to inhale it. Sweet Orange is also great against frustration, tension and anxiety and would help you become calm or have a positive disposition. This way, you can also benefit from it so you and your child can both be happy people.

- **Roman Chamomile**—Roman Chamomile is very effective against tantrums and is also great in helping your child have a calm sleeping time. You can either add this in the bath so it would be easy for you to apply it to your baby or you can put a drop of this on your child's pillow during bedtime so he/she can easily inhale the scent.

- **Sandalwood and Ylang-Ylang**—2 to 3 drops of each of the oils are enough to help in calming your child and making him cheerful and happy.

- **Ylang-Ylang and Mandarin**—2 drops of each are sure to relieve stress and help your baby become calm. This mixture will also help put the baby to sleep easily and you can also be sure that he/she won't have crying fits between sleep.

- **Chamomile and Lavender**—Putting 4 drops each of Lavender and Chamomile on a tissue and placing it under a child's pillow shortly before bedtime is great to sooth babies and children and will also help them fall asleep faster.

- **Lemon**—Lemon acts as a great disinfectant and that's why it is able to clear the air and help you and your child breathe better. You can place this in a diffuser or a piece of cloth for inhalation purposes, or you may choose to add it in water as a dishwashing or cleaning liquid. You may also just keep a spray bottle handy so you can use it to clean your hands easily and to sanitize yourself and your baby.

Chapter 7: Essential Oils for Coughs, Colds and Flu

And of course, what better way to use essential oils than by using them to treat ailments that may easily affect babies and children? Aside from being more affordable than drugs that you can buy from the local pharmacy, essential oils are also great because they are made from natural sources and can also be mixed and matched, depending on what your child's condition is. Here are some of the things that you have to keep in mind with regards to which essential oils are best used against different ailments and how you can use them.

Fight Flu

Even as an adult, it's not very easy to deal with flu. So, just imagine how your child must feel if he/she is experiencing coughs, colds and fever. It's very frustrating for a child to feel this way and as a parent it's hard seeing your kid suffer. So, you need not worry anymore for here's a good mix of essential oils that you can use together to make sure that your child gets rid of flu.

- **Respiratory Comfort**—Spruce, Myrtle, Peppermint, Marjoram, Lavender and Pine
- **Thieves** (don't worry about the name; your child won't be robbed of good health because of this) – Rosemary, Cinnamon Bark, Lemon, Clove, Eucalyptus Radiata
- **Oregano**
- **Lemon**
- **Peppermint**

Why are these oils great against flu? Here are the reasons why:

- Lemon oil is a great disinfectant, as mentioned earlier and since it is a citrus fruit, it works well against inflammation. Lemon also reduces a virus's capability to destroy your child's immune system.
- Peppermint is great for preventing colds, fever or cough. It is naturally cooling and is a great anti-oxidant, too.
- Oregano is known to be a common household treatment for flu. This is the reason why some gardens almost always has oregano in them.
- Thieves are good in controlling the spread of viruses and making sure that your condition does not get worse.
- Thieves are also able to fight cough well. Once taken at the first few signs of cough, it will easily manage the ailment and help you feel better in no time.
- Respiratory Comfort, more commonly known as RC, helps in relieving the pain of sinusitis when applied to one's chest or back or when inhaled using a cloth or diffuser.

You see, the combination of these oils are awesome and can truly help someone feel better.

Ways on how to use these oils:

- You can either breathe in the oils with the help of a cloth or diffuser, or choose to make lozenges or capsules out of them. Breathing the oils is proven to be more effective though as it easily targets the

Amygdala, or the part of the brain that controls emotions, helping one feel calm and better.
- Breathing the oils also help in clearing your airways and help in alleviating the pain that you must be feeling. It also diffuses mucus buildup and helps make your lungs and respiratory system stable and free from damage.
- Boil water in the pot size of your choice and add at least 5 or 6 drops of the oil mixture to it then carry your baby near the pot (but not very near) so he/she will be able to inhale the mixture.
- You may also try directly applying the oils to a baby's skin, most specifically on the back or just near the spine so he/she will easily be able to absorb the oils and so the oils can work on loosening the baby's airways. This way, viruses can easily be fought and the baby can easily feel better, too.
- To alleviate a baby's fever, you could dip a finger in the essential oil mixture and run your finger on the baby's foot. You may also dip the baby's foot in oil, just as long as it's warm and not hot so the oil will be absorbed by the child's skin. If the child finds the scent too strong, you may wrap his/her feet with socks and dip the feet in oil.
- You may also use the oils as spray and spray them on the baby's mouth (provided that they have been diluted) so the baby would easily be able to absorb nutrients that are in the oils.

Using Eucalyptus Oil

Eucalyptus Oil can also be used against coughs and colds. Just place a bowl of water under your child's bed and add 3 drops of Eucalyptus Oil in it. The Eucalyptus Smithi kind is said to be best for children. The steam will then be able to rise around the room and help your child breathe and feel better. Don't use for kids under 3 months old, though.

Chapter 8: Essential Oils for Other Ailments and Health Purposes

Using essential oils against ailments are not just exclusive to coughs, colds and flu. You may also use them for other ailments and health conditions. They are very useful and very effective, plus you won't have a hard time making them, too. Here are some great ideas that you can try and that you should always keep in mind:

Immunity Booster

What better way to make sure that your child's health gets better and that he/she can be safe from ailments than by making sure that your immune system is in tip-top shape? This can easily be done with the help of Lavender and Tea Tree Oil. Both oils are able to produce T-Cells, or the kind of immune cells in a body and stabilizes a child's immune system.

Just mix ½ tsp of unscented shower gel with a drop each of Tea Tree and Lavender Oil then add the said mixture to bath water. Bathe your child with it and you can be sure that he/she will be stronger and better in no time, especially when used daily.

For Digestive Upsets

Pour 2 to 3 drops of Chamomile Oil to Sunflower Oil (as a base) then gently rub the mixture over your child's tummy. Peppermint Oil may be used for children 3 years and older but make sure not to use too much Peppermint Oil as it is quite strong and children may not bear with it well.

A mixture of German Chamomile and Mandarin may also be used against Digestive problems. Just mix them together and rub on your child's tummy 2 or 3 times a day.

For Teething Pain

Add Lavender and Roman Chamomile Oil to your choice of base oil then warm the oil in your palms by rubbing them together. Massage your child's cheeks and jaw-lines with it. Make sure not to put inside a child's mouth or near a child's eyes for safety reasons.

For Diaper Rash

It's very common for babies to suffer from Diaper Rash and it is quite itchy and that's why you have to make sure that you get to help your child in alleviating the pain. By regularly using essential oils during bath time, you can help your child get rid of Diaper Rash. You may also add at least 2 drops of Chamomile Oil to an unscented cream and rub it on your child's butt to get rid of the rashes. 4 drops of tea tree oil can also be used as it is very effective against rashes and insect bites. Lavender Oil is also proven to be very helpful when it comes to getting rid of rashes.

For Earaches

Another common problem that children may experience is earaches. To get rid of this, just massage chamomile oil around the ears and down your child's neck. You may also make use of a mixture of warmed almond oil and 3 drops

Lavender oil and using a medicine dropper to drop it inside a child's ears. This is very cooling and will help get rid of the pain.

For Burns

Essential Oils are also very useful for accidents such as minor burns. After plunging the affected area to cold water, don't forget to apply Lavender oil into it to soothe the pain. Lavender Oil is also effective for severe burns. Chamomile Oil can also be used.

For Foot-aches

Just mix 3 to 5 drops of the essential oil of your choice to warm water and soak your child's foot there for at least 5 minutes. This will soothe the muscles and help alleviate the pain.

Conclusion

Thank you again for purchasing this book!

I hope this book was able to help you to learn more about the benefits of using Essential Oils and what these can do to help make your child feel better and help your child grow up to be a healthy and well-balanced individual.

The next step is to not be afraid to try using essential oils to help your baby feel better and in treating some common ailments that he/she may go through. After all, being a good parent is about learning how to help your child become the best person that he/she can be and that can be done by making sure that he/she is in the pink of health.

Finally, if you enjoyed this book, please take the time to share your thoughts and post a review on Amazon. We do our best to reach out to readers and provide the best value we can. Your positive review will help us achieve that. It'd be greatly appreciated!

Thank you and good luck!

The Ultimate Guide to Vegetable Gardening for Beginners: How to Grow Your Own Healthy Organic Vegetables All Year Round!

http://amzn.to/1lqCCIK

The Ultimate Guide to Raised Bed Gardening for Beginners: How to Grow Flowers and Vegetables in Raised Beds for a Successful Garden

http://amzn.to/1nHY0ry

Greenhouse Gardening for Beginners: How to Grow Flowers and Vegetables Year-Round In Your Greenhouse

http://amzn.to/UEmOr2

Essential Oils Box Set #1: Healing Babies and Children with Aromatherapy for Beginners + Oil Pulling Therapy For Beginners

http://amzn.to/1yZoH0Q

Essential Box Set #2: Carb Cycling For Fast Easy Weight Loss + Walk Your Way to Weight Loss

http://amzn.to/Tu5xiL

Essential Box Set #3: Beauty Products For Beginners + Body Lotions For Beginners

http://amzn.to/1qnVLNQ

Essential Box Set #4: Coconut Oil & Weigh Loss for Beginners & Coconut Oil for Skin Care & Hair Loss

http://amzn.to/1iQQUlN

Essential Oils Box Set #5: Coconut Oil for Skin Care& Hair Loss+ Healing Babies and Children with Aromatherapy for Beginners + Beauty Products For + Body Lotions For Beginners+ Oil Pulling Therapy For Beginners

http://amzn.to/1qGPc6D

Essential Oils Box Set #6: Carb Cycling for Fast Easy Weight Loss+ Oil Pulling Therapy For Beginners + Walk Your Way To Weight Loss + Coconut Oil & Weight Loss For Beginners + Coconut Oil for Skin Care & Hair Loss

http://amzn.to/UXAAoz

Essential Box Set #7: Coconut Oil for Skin Care& Hair Loss + Oil Pulling Therapy For Beginners + Healing Babies and Children with Aromatherapy for Beginners

http://amzn.to/1nUdbg5

Garden Box Set #1: The Ultimate Guide to Raised Bed Gardening for Beginners + The Ultimate Guide to Vegetable Gardening for Beginners + The Ultimate Guide to Companion Gardening for Beginners + Greenhouse Gardening for Beginners + + Container Gardening For Beginners

http://amzn.to/1lZOsse

Gardening Box Set #2: Container Gardening For Beginners + Ultimate Guide to Companion Gardening for Beginners

http://amzn.to/1q4wma5

If the links do not work, for whatever reason, you can simply search for these titles on the Amazon website to find them.

Made in the USA
Middletown, DE
22 December 2015